Deodorants
Easy Recipes For Fresh and Effective Deodorants

Table of Content:

Introduction

When I was still a child I am not experiencing any kinds of bad odor especially on my armpit, it was only when I reached my adolescent stage when I experienced a significant change especially on my metabolism. I began to sweat more which is really a great deal on why I accumulated a bad odor especially on my armpit since then.

I was frustrated and helpless because I have no idea on what to do in battling my bad odor problem. It was really a nightmare for me because I was bullied and I cannot do anything because what they are saying are all true.

I asked my mom on what do I need to do to combat the problem. She told me that I have to cleanse carefully my body especially the armpit when I am taking a bath and apply a deodorant afterward.

I did the routines that my mom advice throughout the years until I became an adult however I am noticing that it has a lot of side-effects not only my skin but also on my overall wellness.

This is the primary reasons why I discovered that the artificial deodorant that I am using is composed of chemicals that are harmful to the health. This is where I had an urge to learn how to make natural deodorant recipes for personal use.

It truly changed my life for the better because it made myself healthier and most importantly free from bad odor. As time passed by, I realized that it wasn't enough for me to keep the knowledge by myself so I decided to share it to you on this book so that you will also have the ability to enjoy the privilege that I have.

Chapter 1 – Why Deodorants Are Important?

Imagine a situation where you enter a public vehicle, let's say a bus or train, or let's say a public place, and then there you are, you suddenly hold your breath or covered your nose for long because of that unwanted smell roaming around the place?

Of course, you know that it came from someone's sweaty underarms and then you might say that "do they even use deodorant?" We all know that it is embarrassing especially if we are on that person's place.

But did you know that the sweat our body produces is odorless or close to it? Then you might ask: "Then where did that bad smell came from?" So let's start with it, our skin pores in the body produce sweat because of the waste that passes through it. The hotter the climate is the more sweat our body produces especially on the warm parts of our bodies, like for example, the underarms.

The bad smell that we all hate doesn't come from the sweat, but from bacteria that is on the sweat. There are a lot of people that use deodorant, and some use them almost every day and continues it for a long period of time where stopping the use if it will never be an option.

There are also other people who don't really need these deodorants or simply does not use them at all, and believe me it is all fine. But for those who use deodorants, they don't really know that the effectiveness of it is just low.

We all know that the deodorant's purpose is to get rid of the body odor in us. And yes it is the main reason and the only reason we have that's why we use deodorants. There is something like deodorant that is called "Antiperspirants", but they function differently.

Antiperspirants keep us from producing body odor thus making us smell fresh, and they stop our sweat glands to produce too much sweat.

But take note that antiperspirants don't really work, I mean, like the deodorant, its effectiveness is low because there will be a time that our body will reject and become immune from the effects of the antiperspirant.

Like you, I am also curious about how exactly deodorants get rid of the bad smell our body have. In all honesty, both things, the deodorant, and antiperspirants are quite complicated. But here today, I'll be listing down some of the effects of deodorants on our body.

1. *Deodorants eliminate those odor-causing bacteria*

Like what I've just said earlier, sweat is almost completely odorless, because there are some studies that proved sweat is nearly odorless. Body odor comes out when the body's bacteria breaks down one of two types of sweat. That only means, the bad smell that we usually produce from excessive sweating doesn't come out right after we sweat for a small amount, and if the sweat doesn't stay too long from your skin.

So all in all, the main idea of deodorant is that they can kill the bacteria that causes bad odor, and that is all.

2. Deodorants do not stop you from sweating

Well, the daily use of deodorants and antiperspirants led some of us to believe that they both work the same way but in reality, they don't. Just like said recently, deodorants keep us from smelling bad, they get rid of the bacteria in the sweat, but they don't stop the sweat glands from producing sweat.

Now, on the other hand, the antiperspirants help to stop the production of excess sweat on the sweat glands in order to get rid of excessive and unwanted sweat, especially on the underarms. So to sum it all up, we put our money on the antiperspirants as they can help you get rid of this annoying extra sweat the same time maintain you smelling fresh, but do keep in mind that they only decrease the sweat glands production of sweat by only 20%.

3. Use of deodorant can change the bacteria in the body

There is a study that stated, the use of deodorants and antiperspirants can change the skin microbiome, meaning that they can somehow affect the bacteria in our body. In this study conducted, there were 17 persons where they are examined for about eight days. The researchers swabbed each of the person's underarms.

The first day of the study, the participants of the study does their standard underarm hygiene routine. Starting the second day up to the sixth, they all stopped using antiperspirants and deodorants. And for the last two days, the seventh and eighth, all of them applied antiperspirants.

As for the final result, it has shown that everyone who participated in the study has an increase of bacteria on their underarms the time they stopped using the antiperspirants and deodorants.

4. Use of deodorant can lead to breast cancer

Some might say that women who use deodorants and antiperspirants every day can increase the chances of them having breast cancer in the future. This may bother some of you, but here is an explanation of why it is not true.

There is a theory that stated, the aluminum in the antiperspirants and the parabens in the deodorants can produce some hormonal effects, estrogen-like. These things can contribute in the growth of breast cancer cells and there are a few numbers of scientific studies that stated there is somehow a connection, but the FDA and the National Cancer Institute does not support this claims.

Now knowing this, we think that you should not be afraid of using deodorants and antiperspirants, why? It is because it is not proven that it can lead to breast cancer, and there are no cases which stated they developed breast cancer because they use deodorants and antiperspirants daily.

There are still studies being conducted about these claims, and as long as it is not yet proven, the use of these products are completely safe.

Why Deodorants are very important for Women in Modern Life?

The use of antiperspirants and deodorants are very high especially on hotter places on earth, for one good reason, people there sweat a lot. And we have our own lives, we have our own jobs, and things we do, physically to be exact, and because of this, we also sweat a lot, like a lot. So how to deal with it?

Grab your deodorant or antiperspirant and your good to go. Well, believe it or not, but these products, the antiperspirants, and deodorants have been running all along the way back to the time of the Ancient Egyptians, well actually it started from them. They experiment with different natural materials to use as scented products for the underarms, one example is cinnamon.

But here in our modern world, most antiperspirants and deodorants contain chemicals in order for a better and likable result.

A lot of us are annoyed when we sweat especially when you are working on an office or a place that is air-conditioned because when the bad odor starts to kick in, it will just spread out in the whole place and the smell will just stay there and somehow will leave a dark spot in your shirt near the underarms. It is just embarrassing, right? But you should know that sweating is actually good for the body.

Sweating is a normal thing that happens in the body, it is a natural way of cooling our bodies when it is hot. So come to think about what happens when you stop it. That is what happens every single time you use an antiperspirant. So it is still important to put the balance on things and try not to use them daily.

Well, having some knowledge about deodorants and antiperspirants can be good, but what if you process more info about it?

Like for example, did you know that we spend almost $18 billion dollars a year for these products, just for the sake of removing bad odors or making your sweat glands stop producing sweat? Come think of that $18 billion dollars. And here, I'll be listing down some of the things that you might not know about antiperspirants and deodorants.

1. Deodorant eliminates bacteria

Well, we all know that the one that causes those bad odors are the bacteria on the sweat, right? So here is the deodorant coming up to save the day. They will keep you smelling good as they eliminate those bacteria that lies in your sweat.

2. The anti-body odor is an old-time trend

Yes, you heard that right. Like said from the previous one up there, the Ancient Egyptians made the first anti-body odor products which are later known as deodorants.

And did you know that the first ever trademarked deodorant is called Mum and was created in 1888, man that is a long time ago. And after 15 years, the first ever antiperspirant came out and it is called Everdry.

3. *Antiperspirants do not really stop the production of sweat.*

This aluminum found in antiperspirants does a good job of stopping the eccrine sweat glands. But it is just 20 percent effective.

4. *Your body can become immune to the antiperspirant you use daily*

Believe it or not but our bodies can adapt to the effects an antiperspirant can do to our sweat glands, and no one knows how can this happen. Some said that the body can find its own way of resisting the effects and starts to produce more sweat on other glands.

A doctor said that it is better to have a variety of brands for deodorants and antiperspirants in order to prevent the body to adapt from its effects.

5. Whether you're a man or woman, deodorant is effective

Do you know that women have more sweat glands than men? Yes, it's true but the cool thing here is men's sweat glands produces more sweat then women do.

Although there are separate products or brands of antiperspirants and deodorants that are specified for men and women, in reality, they are all the same, and all of these "separated" things is just a marketing strategy. And it is funny to think that all of us still falls for this kind of marketing. The only thing that differs is the style and scent of the deodorant.

6. *Some people do not need deodorants*

Well, some may advertise really well that people are still convinced to buy and use deodorants every day. And do you know that most people don't smell bad at all? Yes, it is all true. And some people are simply lucky because they naturally don't smell bad at all because of their genes.

7. No one really knows where those yellow stains came from

Not even the ones who make deodorants and antiperspirants and not even the scientists know why are there yellow stains left in the underarms when they use deodorants and antiperspirants.

But the main thing here is that some theorize that it came from the aluminum compounds which can be seen on antiperspirants as they have certain chemical reactions with the sweat, shirt or the skin.

And according to some research, the best way to get rid of these yellow stains is just to simply avoid buying and using aluminum-based antiperspirants.

8. *You can produce your own deodorant and antiperspirant*

Isn't that amazing that you can improvise or somehow create your own deodorant and antiperspirant right at your own home! Well, there are certain things or ingredients needed in order to make one.

The bright side of making your own deodorant or antiperspirant is that it is very easy to do, and for the brighter side of it, it can cost you less or nothing at all because they are purely natural, all you need is some certain oil and extracts together with its antibacterial compounds which can add up in removing those unwanted bad smell from your underarm.

Chapter 2 – Artificial Versus Natural Deodorants

Starting with this topic, I'll give you the things you must know in order to understand what is in between these two types of deodorants and how they completely differ from each other. So first things first, what is an artificial deodorant? It is obvious, right?

An artificial deodorant is made up of chemicals and partly natural ingredient. On the other hand, is the All-Natural Deodorant, well we also know that this is very obvious, it all tells it by its name. These deodorants are all made from natural and organic materials or ingredients in order to make those scented anti-bacterial bad odor removing deodorants.

Now that I gave you a head start in today's topic, I will be listing down the things you must know why you should switch from artificial deodorant into natural ones. But first why?

In reality, we can use those artificially made deodorants in general but you might want to know that these deodorants don't work at all for some people, because sometimes their body resists these product's effectiveness.

You might be one of these people and in order for you to have a working deodorant product, you might want to try being all-natural in this situation, what I mean is start researching about certain ingredients you can use in making your own natural deodorant that will perfectly work on your body and can adapt on your sweat glands. So now I will be listing down the reasons why you should use natural deodorants than artificial ones.

1. *Artificial deodorants do contain ingredients that can be harmful to your health*

So here we are again talking about the risks of using deodorants and antiperspirants. There is a study that proved, using aluminum-based antiperspirants can increase the chance of having an Alzheimer's disease by 60 percent.

And yet the theory of increasing the chance of having breast cancer by using aluminum-based antiperspirants are here again although this claim about cancer is not yet proven, why not just become safe and try to change your old aluminum-based antiperspirant into a not aluminum based one right?

2. Natural deodorants have ingredients that are good for your body

There are natural deodorants that contain charcoal on it, and for you to know, it is not only the natural deodorants that use charcoal but also other cosmetic products. So what does this charcoal do exactly?

It helps absorbs moisture more than you can think of and wait for it, the best part is when charcoal is ingested, it can help you with gastrointestinal problems, can you believe that? Can your recent artificial deodorant do that? There are some plant-based deodorants that can help your underarms to stay fresh and smooth. These ingredients are olive oil, clay-rich in mineral, and Shea butter.

They help make your underarms to become smooth and irritation free. When your underarms do not irritate from the artificial products you use, underarm shaves can last longer. And there are some other ingredients that can help smoothen out razor burns and shrink pores.

The good thing about these natural deodorants is that they don't block the pores in our skin unlike what the antiperspirants do. What these natural deodorant do is they let the good bacteria do their own thing on your skin which is to help lessen the odor.

Because like said previously, it is not the sweat that causes the bad odor, the odor only comes out when the bacteria mixes with your sweat. That's why using natural deodorants can help you get rid of this bacteria, making you smell good.

3. *Does detoxification happen whenever you switch from artificial to natural deodorant?*

There is one statement that said they don't believe in a detoxification period once you switched from artificial to natural deodorant. They stated that once you use the natural one, it will immediately work on the spot.

But for those first timers in using natural deodorants, they must understand that the effectiveness of it still depends on a person's way of living, the food he or she eats and his or her daily physical activities and many more. You must also take note that an aluminum-free deodorant doesn't stop sweat at all.

Those only with ingredients that are safe for you will just help stop the bad odor but they won't keep you dry for the whole day, I mean, they won't keep you dry at all. Just don't stop the sweating, it is not harmful and like said, the sweat is not the one that causes the bad odor, but the bacteria mixed on it. In reality, sweating is a sign that your body is healthy. Don't you want that?

Based on my study, some said that the best way to make the most out of your deodorant is to balance how much you use it. Some people claimed that one or two swipes of deodorants helped them stayed odorless the whole day. And please keep in mind that unlike the artificial deodorants, natural ones only need small amounts to be applied to your underarm in order to work.

Things You Must Know about the Natural and Artificial Deodorants

Of course, you are here for a reason, and that is to know how does these two differ? What are their advantages on each other, disadvantages? And yeah, you are finding the one that will best suit your situation, or in other words, you are finding what product will work best for your body.

It is common for us that we always find precautionary measures in order to be safe from the products that we are going to use.

Well, in this part of the article, I'll be answering down the most common questions asked by people about natural deodorants and artificial deodorants. Stay tuned, you might find the answer you've been looking for here.

1. *Are deodorants and antiperspirants the same?*

For a simpler explanation, the antiperspirants work is to stop the sweat glands from producing sweat, well in reality, not stop at all but reduces its production, while the deodorant, on the other hand, stops that annoying bad odor that lingers around whenever your underarms sweat. Although antiperspirants are also deodorants, not all deodorants are antiperspirants. Think of it as an additional feature for deodorant.

2. *So which one stands out?*

So starting off, antiperspirants stop our sweat glands from sweating right?

I believe that you know sweating is a part of the body's process, and it is a sign of healthiness. Sweating is the body's natural way of ventilation. A doctor said that if you don't sweat (naturally), it is a sign that your body can't or doesn't release the toxins inside that can be harmful to us or it is that you are having a bad metabolism.

The aluminum compound in the antiperspirant is an actual aluminum, and it is the most bothering ingredient this product has. So how does this work basically? These small aluminum compounds find their way to block those cells and pores on the skin thus making it look like your sweat glands stopped from producing sweat.

The use of aluminum products like utensils and other stuff has become controversial over the years, and I think that it goes the same with the deodorant. We must stop using aluminum-based antiperspirants. Because long-term use of this aluminum based product can cause serious damage to our tissues.

There is a study that shows aluminum are neurotoxins and can contribute massively to the production of breast cancer cells (the reason why aluminum-based antiperspirants are linked to breast cancer). Not just that, but it can also make the chances of having an Alzheimer's disease high and can cause toxicity in the liver.

Someone said that the use of antiperspirants depends on the person's need. Although the use of antiperspirants is commonly linked with breast cancer, one person stated that the aluminum compounds in the antiperspirants are too small for our body to absorb it completely and cause serious damage inside.

Because studies are still being conducted about the link of antiperspirants on breast cancer, if they are really connected, or if that antiperspirants really cause estrogen to change causing breast cancer cells to increase in amount.

But in order for you to find out what's best for your skin, I suggest that you look at the ingredients of the product you are going to buy.Look if there are common components that can cause skin irritation, these ingredients, for example, are the following propylene glycol, formaldehyde, geraniol, linalool, carboxaldehyde, benzyl salicylate.

And if you are deciding on what type of deodorant to buy, if it's a roll-on, stick, cream or spray. I suggest using the first three and try to avoid sprays, why? Deodorants are meant for skin, not the lungs. It is better to be safe.

3. *Any tips on how can I switch from one product to another?*

Well, made up your mind already in changing up your old deodorant? But do keep in mind that before starting a new one you must know that it will change your body care routine.

Some of the natural deodorant users suggest that you detoxify your underarms first right after you get rid of your old deodorant. And I also believe that this is essential, it is because the detoxification will remove the excess chemicals your old deodorant had left on your underarms.

Think of this as a new fresh start, then right after you've detoxified your underarms, you can now start with your new deodorant brand. There is a simple mask you can make right at your house for this underarm detoxification, all you need is to mix up these ingredients with water: bentonite clay, apple cider, and vinegar.

Well if you are not a fan of that detoxification thing, don't worry. There is a statement that said our body has a natural way of detoxification, and yes I think you already know what that is already.

Yes, of course, sweating. Being part of the natural processes of the body, there is no need to worry from chemicals harming you.

When you already started to use your all new natural deodorant and noticed that it is not working at all, you might want to try to exfoliate your underarms once a week. To do these, all you need is a washcloth then mix it up with oat flour and then unscented oil like coconut oil, then you're good to go.

Now that some of your questions are answered, now I will be listing down the reasons why you should avoid artificial deodorants and antiperspirants and start using natural deodorants now. Is it already obvious that all thing that is natural can benefit us a lot than those with chemical. But why do we keep on patronizing this artificial product? Is it because it is easy to buy?

Saves us time in preparing our own because these artificial ones are pre-made already? Yes, these reasons are also beneficial, but come think of this, is it beneficial for your own health? For me, I don't think so.That is why the best way to stay healthy, fresh and odor free, is to get rid of these artificial deodorants and antiperspirants and start using pure natural deodorants and antiperspirants.

Don't mind the time for preparation and the ingredients, because in the end it will be all worth it. So here are the reasons why you should give up your present artificial deodorant and antiperspirant.

1. Artificial deodorants and antiperspirants contain harmful ingredients

Yes that is right. It is mentioned a lot in this article, especially the antiperspirant having aluminum on its ingredients. So it is better to stay away from these chemical based products in order to reduce or the best, completely avoid complications in your body.

2. Natural deodorants don't contain any aluminum

Although artificial antiperspirants stop the sweat glands from sweating because of the aluminum ions that blocks it. Natural deodorants, on the other hand, work in a very different and safer way.

There are compounds in the natural deodorants that help absorb wetness in the underarms effectively, these are plant-based powders and sodium bicarbonate or also known as baking soda.

3. *The scent of natural deodorants are also natural and chemical free*

What does this one mean? Artificial deodorants' scents contain a lot of chemicals in order to create that particular scent.

So imagine now the chemicals that flow right into your body. With the natural deodorants, it is all different, as it provides scent coming from essential oils which are all purely natural.

Chapter 3 – Amazing All-Natural Deodorant Recipes

We are close at the end of this article, and before we part ways, I would like to say thank you for staying until this part, so let us not waste some time, and let's get through this.

Now, I will be listing down recipes that can help you make natural deodorants in your own house. I bet that you've read all the things that natural deodorant do? It is all beneficial rather than those artificial ones, right?

And I think that we must be concerned about the products we are using that is why I suggest that you do the natural ones as they don't contain harmful chemicals that artificial deodorants have. There is this ingredient in artificial deodorants called parabens, these include methyl, ethyl, propyl, benzyl, and butyl.

These ingredients are commonly found on the artificial deodorants you are using, and man, that is a lot of chemicals. And there are claims that these chemicals are linked also with breast cancer and other various diseases.

Here are some of the harmful chemicals or ingredients on artificial deodorants that you should avoid:

1. *Parabens (methyl, ethyl, propyl, benzyl, and butyl) - these chemicals are linked with breast cancer and other diseases.*
2. *Aluminum Compounds- often found in antiperspirants, these metallic materials are also linked with breast cancer.*
3. *Silica- These ingredients or chemicals are harmful to the body as they can contribute to cancer and allergies.*
4. *Triclosan- This ingredient is linked with cancer and skin irritations.*
5. *Talc- a chemical that is also linked with cancer.*

6. *Propylene Glycol- these chemicals are linked with liver and kidney problems and also allergic reactions.*
7. *Steareth-n- it is also linked with cancer.*

For the natural deodorant ingredients, here they are:

Homemade Deodorant for a Sensitive Skin

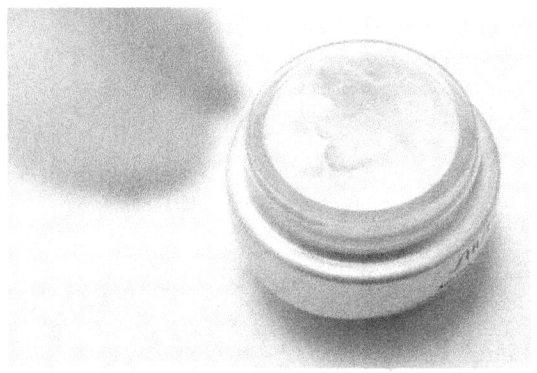

Ingredients:

3/4 cup arrowroot powder/non-GMO cornstarch
1/4 cup baking soda
4-6 tbsp. melted coconut oil

Procedure:

1. In a bowl, mix up the baking soda cornstarch or arrowroot powder
2. Then add up four tablespoons of melted coconut oil then mix. Keep on adding coconut oil until desired consistency is achieved.
3. Put the mixture into a jar with a tight cover.

Shea Butter Deodorant

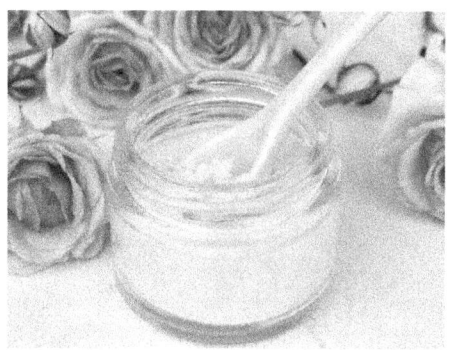

Ingredients:

3 tbsp. coconut oil
3 tbsp. baking soda
2 tbsp. shea butter
2 tbsp. arrowroot (optional) or organic cornstarch
Essential oils (optional)

Procedure:

1. Start by melting the Shea butter and coconut oil in a boiler over medium heat or you can just combine the coconut oil and the Shea butter in a glass jar with a cover then place it over in a pan with water until it melts.
2. Remove from heat then add up the arrowroot or if you don't have arrowroot, add more baking soda.
3. Then add up the essential oils then put all the mixture in a glass container. Don't need to the refrigerator. But it is up to you if you want to put it in the fridge, just to make it hard quickly.

Essential Oil Deodorant

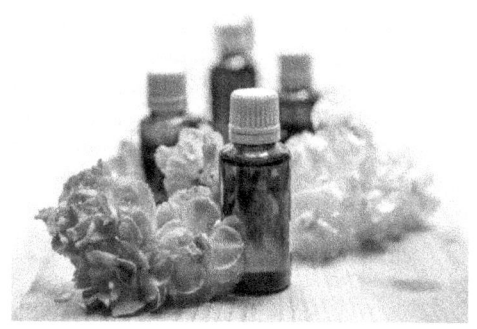

Ingredients:

2 1/2 tbsp. unrefined coconut oil

2 1/2 tbsp. unrefined shea butter

1/4 cup arrowroot starch/flour

2 tbsp. baking soda

6 drops lavender essential oil

6 drops grapefruit essential oil

2 drops tea tree essential oil (optional)

Procedure:

1. In a bowl or jar, put the coconut oil and Shea butter then place the bowl or jar in a medium pan.

2. Add water to the pan, just the right amount to surround the jar or bowl then boil it.

3. As it boils, continue to stir the coconut oil and Shea butter until it melts down.

4. Then right after, place it in separate jars (it is up to you what size) then put it in the fridge so that it will become hard quickly.

5. Make sure to keep the cover on when not in use.

Herbal Deodorant Spray

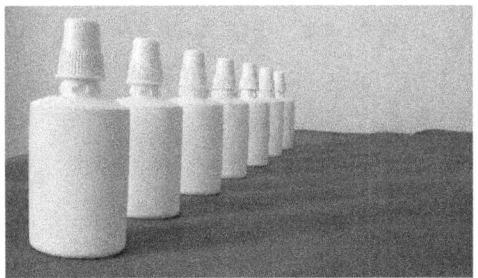

Ingredients:

1¼ cup 80 proof vodka

¼ cup sage leaves

¼ cup thyme leaves

¼ cup lavender buds

Peel of 1 lime or lemon

Essential oils:

Sage (6 drops)

Lavender (4 drops)

Tea tree (3 drops)

Patchouli (3 drops), and either lemongrass or

lime(3 drops) per quarter-cup spray bottle

½ tsp. colloidal silver per quarter cup spray bottle,

optional

Procedure:

1. In a pint-size jar, measure the herbs and citrus peels.
2. Pour vodka then cover it.
3. Keep the jar in a place where you can always find it, shake it once a day for about a month.
4. When the mixture is ready, funnel the liquid into a spray bottle.
5. Then add up the essential oil for fragrance.
6. Place the drained herbs somewhere you can find it until you are ready to use it again for another mixture.

7. Shake the spray bottle to mix up all the ingredients inside and not letting it only sit right on the top of the bottle.
8. Then you are good to go.

We've come the end of this article and I hope that you've learned a lot about deodorants and antiperspirants. This should give you the knowledge on what to use and how to use them.

To summarize them all, there are certain chemicals found in the ingredients of artificial deodorants and antiperspirants that can be extremely harmful to your health. So it is better to use the artificial ones as they give you the same results in a more safe way and much better.

Conclusion

There you have it, I hope that you have learned a lot from the wonderful deodorant recipes that are included in this book. Do not delay the action now and stop using artificial deodorants and starting switching to the natural ones that are included in the recipes that I mentioned on the previous chapters.

We therefore conclude that those recipes will bring us hundred folds of benefits that is why it is really necessary to put it on your daily routines. Be like me, because based on experience those recipes really improved myself not only my body odor, health, but also my confidence.

So if you want to improve your life for the better then take an action now. I wish you all the best in life!